T0005289

THE SKIN SAVVY

WOMAN OF COLOR

TERRY M. PURDIE

THE SKIN SAVVY
WOMAN OF COLOR

AN EASY GUIDE TO ACHIEVING PHENOMENAL SKIN
THROUGH PHENOMENAL CARE

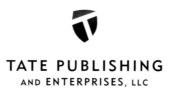

TATE PUBLISHING
AND ENTERPRISES, LLC

Published by Tate Publishing & Enterprises, LLC
127 E. Trade Center Terrace | Mustang, Oklahoma 73064 USA
1.888.361.9473 | www.tatepublishing.com

Tate Publishing is committed to excellence in the publishing industry. The company reflects the philosophy established by the founders, based on Psalm 68:11,
"The Lord gave the word and great was the company of those who published it."

Book design copyright © 2013 by Tate Publishing, LLC. All rights reserved.
Cover design by Joel Uber
Interior design by Honeylette Pino

Published in the United States of America

ISBN: 978-1-62563-842-7
1. Health & Fitness / Body Cleansing & Detoxification
2. Health & Fitness / Women's Health
13.08.08

DEDICATION

To the honor and glory of the Lord Almighty
and to my Savior Jesus Christ

ACKNOWLEDGMENTS

To my Lord Jesus who gave me the desire to serve people through skin care and presented me with the gift of wisdom, knowledge, and an understanding heart to do so. It is by his grace and power without which this book would not have been possible.

To my husband, Steve, thank you for helping with the shows on the road, the driving, finances, packing and unpacking, set up and break down, painting, fit-ups, and moving. Thank you for allowing me to pursue my vision. You were there at the beginning of this twenty-year journey, and I appreciate everything you've done and continue to do to support me. Thank you for your love and pride in my accomplishments. I love you very much.

To my beautiful children—Micah, Marcus, Jasmine, and Jordan—I love you so much. Mega thanks and a big mommy hug for your supreme support (the product launch, website, production, and the magazine). Thank you for cheering me on. You guys are the best waiters/waitress, hosts/hostess, test models, sales team, and packagers ever! Marcus, thank you for your special help and the extra time you put in with everything from marketing to pursuing clients and building the brand. Thanks for all your input, diligence, hard work, and prayers of which you excitedly and willing offered and for being my VP of sales and marketing. Thank you for believing in and catching my vision.

To Darius and Jean Ferrell (Daddy and Momma) for the encouragement, teaching me that I can do all things through Christ, and for making me understand that I am a wonderful unique individual that God has created, and therefore I am someone very important. Thank you, Mom and Dad, for the time you spent listening (and listening!), for your spot-on advice, and for your love and care for me. Thank you for believing in me.

To my beautiful sisters and brother who call on me for skin care advice and value my expertise, thanks guys for appreciating my talents and telling others about me.

To my clients and friends, I thank you that I am not just someone with a business, but you have made me a part of your family sharing your photos, celebrations, and sometimes, life's setbacks with me. I feel honored to be so much a part of your lives.

To my best friends Linda and Patty, you guys encourage me so much and make me feel like I am the smartest person in the world—what a feeling! Patty, I miss you, but we will meet again when we all get together with our Lord!

To my fellow lady entrepreneurs, thank you for the encouragement, support, networking, professional advice, and pep talks. Kim, Lonna, Dion, my prayer is for your continued success and promotion.

May the Lord bless and keep you all. May he cause his face to shine upon you; may his peace and grace be upon you is my prayer. I love you all. Thank you for blessing me so.

TABLE OF CONTENTS

INTRODUCTION

To every woman who has been frustrated with her skin, I feel you.

To every individual who has not liked the reflection in the mirror, I see you.

To every soul that has asked questions but seemingly has not received answers, I hear you.

To every wounded heart hounded by low self-esteem, I know you.

I say to you all—you are beautiful and wonderfully made. Let me minister to you.

We've all heard that beauty is only skin-deep, but ugliness goes clean to the bone! I'm here to tell you that beauty is not just skin-deep, but radiates out from deep within the soul and spirit. Every individual has a beautiful person inside of them. When you let the beauty on the inside dominate, it permeates your outward person.

You are a rare specimen. Take a mirror and study your features. Observe the curve of your brows, lips, and cheekbones. Notice the spacing of your eyes and lashes. Turn your head from side to side and take in your jawline. What do you see?

I can tell you what you see—someone fearfully and wonderfully made! (Psalms 139:14)

Understand this about yourself. God made you special. There is no one in this world that is exactly like you. He made you the individual that you are. When you leave this earth, you will become extinct. There is no one who can replace you. God put the biological factors together that produced you. He personally selected your skin tone, hair color and texture, color of your eyes. He "made thee and formed thee from the womb" (Isaiah 44:2). He designed you! He thought enough of you to make you into his own image "Let us make man in our image, after our likeness… So God created man in his own image…male and female created He them…" (Genesis 1:26–27). The very hairs of your head are numbered (Matthew 10:30), even the gray ones. You are valuable to him "… ye are of more value than many sparrows" (Matthew 10:31).

It would seem that if we mean this much to God, we ought to at least value ourselves equally as well. He doesn't and cannot lie. His word is truth. Know that you are someone worth investing in, valuing, and treasuring. This is what it's all about, investing in *you*!

Take a journey with me to discover the real you. Let me enrich your mind, dispel myths, deliver truth, and enhance your personal well-being. We'll trek through the mélange of skin care products to a civilized culture in the world of "me." On the way, you'll grow to skin fitness. You'll be able to choose the correct products to achieve proper balance, intelligently converse with your esthetician (skin care therapist) about your skin and understand what he/she does as a professional. You'll get information that will help you obtain a complexion that will glow from head to toe.

With that said, turn the page! Get comfortable, grab a highlighter or two, and get ready to devote some time to you. What are you waiting for? Enjoy!

WHAT ABOUT ME?

In the Beginning, There Was Skin...

Get focused. Part of what makes you specifically you is the matter that holds the appendages of hair and nails in place that carries the wonderfully varied pigment tones that grace this planet. If you hadn't noticed, your skin covers you from the crown of your head to the soles of your feet. It is one of the components that makes you distinctly you. Good and consistent care of this covering will keep you looking good for many years to come. An integral part of this consistent care includes providing the necessary nutrients for optimal performance of all bodily functions. Proper nutrition is what fuels the body and causes it to perform at its best. Nutrition nourishes your cells which forms the tissues that organs are made of. The organs in turn comprise the different systems of the body—respiratory, excretory, circulatory, nervous, skeletal, muscular, endocrine, digestive, and integumentary. These systems enable your body to function. Proper diet is reflected in your skin, hair, and nails. If you're not properly taking care of your body, it's going to affect how you look and feel.

The skin is both a tissue and an organ and is part of the integumentary system. It varies in thickness—being thickest on the soles of the feet and palms of the hands and is at its thinnest on the eyelids. It is the epithelial tissue—the protective covering of the body. As an organ, it regulates body heat and houses sweat and oil glands, sensory receptors (heat, cold, sensation/touch, and pain), hair and nails, not to mention an assortment of vessels, nerve endings, and such. This marvelous piece of machinery also serves as a barrier or the first line of defense against microorganisms that would seek to invade the body and cause sickness and disease.

The information above by itself should be enough to convince us take care of our covering.

As a tissue, the skin is somewhat elastic and has the ability to repair and renew itself (usually) under normal conditions. The surface is slightly acidic, which plays a major role in its duties to maintain the healthy integrity of the body. This slightly acidic barrier acts as a deterrent to harmful organisms that come into contact with it or try to enter the body through it. In its normal state, it is free from disease (obviously), pliable and soft, slightly moist (good hydration) with a good texture (minimal bumps or raised areas, etc.). It cools the body when overheated through perspiration and tries to warm it by producing goose bumps to generate heat. It protects the internal organs, muscles, vessels, and bones.

It is so amazing that we have this wonderful covering that takes care of us as long as we take care of it!

Black (or Brown) Don't Crack...

One of the most frequent comments made among people of color is "black don't crack," and for whatever reasons, many people feel that special care is not needed to keep the skin in proper condition. As we mentioned earlier, the skin (all skin, no matter the color) functions as a tissue and an organ. Skin of color does have some traits or characteristics that give it somewhat of an advantage over a more fair complexion; however, the blessing is a double-edged sword. The many things that are in its favor are also the same things that if taken for granted, destroy it.

Let's get back to our black don't crack theory. Back in the day, when your mother and grandmother were younger, they lived in a totally different environment than you. This is true as well for your great-grandmother and so forth. Most likely there were not a lot of preservatives and additives in food. People tended home gardens or frequently bought fresh produce from local farmers. Some of us may remember a few chickens in grandma's yard and having fresh bird for supper. (Okay, so that may be way back for some of us).

Cars were in use, but not nearly as many as have been on the road in the last four decades. From the early 1900s to now, can you imagine how many cars are on the road now? Exhaust fumes and other industry excretions were not in abundance comparatively speaking, so poor air quality was not nearly as bad as it is in some places today. Water, milk, juices, and even soda were a lot different. Water certainly may have been a little more pure and it wasn't bottled either!

All of these factors come into play when we speak of how momma or grandma's skin looks. Consider what they consumed. From today's dietary standpoint, quite a few items on the menu may not be the best thing to eat on a regular basis. In retrospect, there was not the same type of exposure to chemicals experienced by the older generations. It would probably be safe to assume that there was a minimal absorption of agents into bodily systems. However, with the surge of modern food packaging technologies and increased use of pesticides and other chemicals, newer generations are faced with different skin and health concerns than our ancestors. Why do you think everyone is on this organically grown kick now? It's because that's how it was done years ago, and someone finally decided there was nothing wrong with it. Think about the air and water quality. These affected the quality of the food, the nourishment the body received.

Grandma did not experience the cumulative effect of environmental stress on her skin like you do. There was hardly any at all. Lifestyles were slower paced. People took time to relax and to enjoy life more. The weekend was really "a weekend," folks rarely worked on Saturday and Sunday. In fact, most everything was closed by six o'clock Saturday evening and absolutely nothing opened on Sunday! There has been a considerable change of lifestyle with each generation. You've heard of free radicals? Eighty years ago, was there ever such a thing heard of in the skin care realm? A generation is considered to be forty years. If this is the case, we are only talking two generations ago, or even to three generations, as families go today. There are acids, dirt, oils, and bacteria in the air that your skin comes into contact with on a daily basis. Combine this with stress and the sun, and there's another party entirely going on. Are you beginning to understand now how these factors weigh heavily in the balance when comparing generations?

Many are the advances in technology that our ancestors did not have that seemingly provide us with the latest and greatest in skin care. But when you consider that they did not have a lot of the problems we are consumed with, does it really matter? All things are relative. Grandma is grandma, and you are you.

With these things in mind, let's focus on how your skin is today. Without getting extremely technical and giving a full course on the histology of the skin, let's just talk about what makes skin of color, "skin of color." Skin of color contains melanin—the pigment that gives it color. All skin contains roughly the same amount of melanocytes (these produce the pigment). The size, distribution, and number of this pigment in the skin layers determine an individual's skin tone. People of color tend to have larger melanocyte cells and have a more even distribution of these cells through the upper skin layers. It is believed that this cellular ingredient reduces the effects of ultraviolet damage to DNA. Because of this coloring, an individual has *limited* natural sun protection, which provides a slower or reduced rate at which signs of premature aging begin to manifest. Hence, natural tanning is a defense mechanism by the body to protect the vulnerable cells in the deeper layers of the skin. It is also believed that melanin absorbs free radicals and this is another reason that darker skin tones do not show signs of aging as much as lighter tones do. Certainly this is an advantage.

Aha, you say? Black *doesn't* crack. But wait, there's only limited sun protection, and the rate at which signs of aging begin to show is reduced. Not complete protection and no signs of aging. Do not assume or take for granted that your darker complexion is a shield of armor. Darker skin can burn and experience damage from the harmful effects of UV rays (more on that in another chapter). As a result, signs of aging do occur even if at a slower rate.

Okay. So what are other characteristics of darker skin? Skin of color, when traumatized, tends to hyperpigment or leave areas that are darker than the surrounding skin on the surface resulting in an uneven skin tone and dark blotches. (Hyperpigmentation does take place in lighter skin tones). When blemishes are picked, a breakout or rash has occurred, or a wound has healed, it is not uncommon to find that the healed tissue has turned darker than the surrounding tissue.

Skin disorders in darker complexions are sometimes harder to diagnose and may continue for a long period before being treated. This is a major problem in diagnosing skin cancer, the rate of which among people of color is increasing steadily. A delay in treatment of this or some other disorder may in some cases prove fatal. Interestingly, people of color are being found to have cancers in places not usually reported in lighter complexioned counterparts. These places include the soles of the feet and palms of the hands.

So what are we trying to say? Because of its sensitivity to trauma, black skin or any skin leaning toward a darker hue is very vulnerable and must be treated with extreme care. Black (skin) does crack, just not as fast as others and in different ways. The everyday environmental, emotional, and physical stresses that your skin goes through compounded with diets filled with preservatives, toxins, high sodium, and few vitamins and minerals sets your skin up for a dull, unhealthy lackluster existence. Dryness, inflammation, breakouts, and uneven color abound. If the skin is not receiving proper nutrients, hydration, UV protection, and good practical hygiene, it will not thrive. The cumulative effects of these properties are greatly increased and continue to rise since grandma was a young girl, and without a doubt, only grow more severe over time. What conclusion can we draw from this? No matter what color the skin, exceptional care is always needed!

What Type of Skin Condition Do I Have?

It is important for each individual to find out their current skin condition. We're not speaking of genetic factors that you cannot change, which is your skin type (like the color, aside from hyperpigmentation and pore size), but its condition. Your skin condition (oiliness, dryness, etc.) is what you will work on. It is to your advantage to seek out the professional advice of an esthetician and to have a thorough skin analysis conducted. In the meantime, here's a list provided below. As you can see, there are several categories to choose from. This is just a general guideline to help you determine which condition you might fall into, a pretty good idea of where to begin at least. If you do not have access to an esthetician, you can use this guide to help you in your selection of products for your skin. Again, this is a guide; it is not all encompassing (no medical disorders listed), and every individual will be different. So never set your standards by what someone else's skin is doing, but understand that you can achieve your own goals of clarity of skin with consistence and persistence.

No matter what your skin condition, proper skin care with the correct product can produce dramatic results.

Possible Skin Condition	Characteristics
Normal	Free of blemishes, slightly elastic, slightly moist to touch, soft and balanced. Not prone to breakouts.
Normal/Dry	Combination – May have dry areas, such as on the cheeks, between the eyes, etc., but basically fine everywhere else. Not usually prone to more than hormonal breakouts.
Normal/Oily	Combination – Usually experiences oiliness in the T-Zone (forehead to nose to chin) and has breakout limited to those areas. Cheeks tend to be only slightly oily or normal and somewhat balanced. The opposite may also be true in that the cheeks are oilier than the forehead, nose and chin.
Oily	Excess oil experienced in all areas. Prone to mild breakout may increase due to hormonal changes. Experiences shine and oily feeling throughout the day. Just a few blemishes. Use of harsh cleansers can exacerbate condition.
Acneic	Experiences excess oil and shine throughout the day with moderate to severe blemishes (with pustules) and blackheads. May seek medical help and prescription drugs to control breakout.
Sensitive/Sensitized	Prone to react to a variety of stimulus such as medicines, environmental factors, product ingredients, emotions or foods. Typically becomes red and inflamed when triggered by an allergen. May be dry or oily and itchy. May breakout in small rashes where contact made with allergen. May itch in hot and cold weather.
Mature or premature aging	Prone to wrinkles and fine lines due to lack of sun protection and/or the natural aging process. May be dry and lack hydration. Usually not prone to breakout, except during hormonal changes (menopause), but can show signs of sensitivity. Lacks elasticity. Complexion may be dull and uneven with dark areas of hyperpigmentation. Also, in lighter tones, skin may have a yellow or sallow appearance.
Oil Dry	Typically has dull slightly ashen appearance. Shows signs of flaking in different areas. Feels tight. May itch and flake excessively. Due to inactivity or sluggishness of oil glands.
Moisture Dry (Dehydrated)	Skin feels dry to the touch. May feel rough in the lip area and have a chapped appearance. When stretched, fine white lines appear on the skin. Prone to fine lines due to lack of moisture, usually a result of inadequate water consumption and/or proper moisture protection.

WHY CUSTOMIZED SKIN CARE IS IMPORTANT

What Is an Esthetician? How Does an Esthetician Help? Why Do I Care?

An esthetician is a person educated and trained in the art of skin care. They operate in either a nonclinical capacity (salons, skin care centers, day or resort spas) or in medispas (licensed physician is on staff) and administer advanced treatments to cleanse condition and care for the skin. They also perform facial massage, body treatments, and makeup application. They do not prescribe medication for acne or any other skin-related medical condition, but may work in conjunction with a dermatologist to care for the skin while a condition heals. They are not psychic and all-knowing. Most states require that an esthetician receive a professional education and licensing. When you visit a good skin care center for treatment, they will analyze your skin to assess its condition and recommend an appropriate treatment. During an analysis, the esthetician is looking for key indications or signs of imbalance (dry patches, excess oil, uneven texture, black/whiteheads, sun damage, hyperpigmentation, etc). It is the role of the esthetician to educate and assist you to help determine your condition based on the findings of their analysis, as well as provide results-oriented treatments. As they are not able to diagnose medical conditions, you will be referred to a dermatologist if something out of the ordinary is going on with your skin. They are very knowledgeable and an excellent resource to obtain information.

Your Customized Care

As you've already seen, there are many different skin conditions. It would be illogical to believe that one product by itself could adequately address all skin conditions with regard to specific needs. It's crucial, therefore, to have at least a little basic knowledge about your skin before you purchase your skin care regimen. Again, an esthetician is of great help in these matters, but knowing about these things yourself is certainly to your benefit and helps you converse intelligently with regard to your needs.

For example, let's say you know that your skin is oily and prone to breakouts; a formulation for dry skin would not be of any use to you. A number of dry skin formulas simulate oil production. That wouldn't be a good thing for an already oily skin. Equally absurd would be to purchase a formulation that addresses oily skin and apply it to dry skin. You'll end up drying the skin further. So don't just pick up any old thing. We're talking about your skin! Treat it with care and take the time to select carefully. Ask questions. The only stupid questions are those that aren't asked before it's too late.

Following a professional program customized just for you will make a world of difference in the appearance and condition of your skin. The benefits accrued by selecting the correct formulation are manifested in proper clearing of the skin, hydration (moisture retention), sufficient balance of oils, and overall healing. When we remain persistent and consistent in pursuing our skin care goals, then we are rewarded with a beautiful complexion.

There are other factors that will play a role in your skin's health and appearance and need to be taken into consideration. After identifying the condition that best describes your skin, answer the questions in the table below. This additional information can be used to further investigate possible causes of trouble spots and may give assistance in how to help resolve the condition. Answer each question carefully. You'll want to relay this information to your esthetician also.

Are you currently under a physician's care? Are you currently taking any medication?
Do you have any allergies? (please list)
Do you have high blood pressure or diabetes? ☐Y ☐N   Are you HIV Positive?   ☐Y ☐N
Are you pregnant?   ☐Y ☐N   Have you had a hysterectomy?   ☐Y ☐N
Are you going through menopause? ☐Y ☐N
Are you using oral contraceptives ☐Y ☐N
Do you exercise regularly? ☐Y ☐N
Do you smoke?   ☐Y ☐N   Do you consume alcohol? ☐Y ☐N
How many caffeinated beverages to you consume daily? _____
How much water do you drink daily?   ☐ Less than 16 oz.   ☐ 16 – 32 oz.   ☐ 32 – 64 oz.   ☐ More than 64 oz.
Do you take vitamins? ☐Y ☐N   Are you dieting? ☐Y ☐N
How often do you experience breakouts?   ☐often   ☐sometimes   ☐rarely
Are breakouts in the form of blackheads/white heads? Both?
Are you being treated for acne?   ☐no ☐mild case ☐moderate case ☐severe case   Excessive oiliness? ☐Y ☐N
Do you experience dryness, redness or tightness? ☐Y ☐N
Do you notice any redness occurring from heat, cold or wind exposure? ☐Y ☐N
Does your skin itch and burn and become easily inflamed? ☐Y ☐N
Do you use sunscreen? ☐Y ☐N
Are you using any of the following? Check all that apply: ☐cleanser   ☐soap & water   ☐toner   ☐nothing   ☐moisturizer   ☐exfoliant/scrub   ☐masque   ☐eye treatment cream   ☐night cream
How often do you cleanse your skin?   ☐ Twice daily   ☐ Once daily   ☐Other

First and foremost your overall wellness has to be accounted for. This is true when beginning a fitness program or starting a specialized diet.

Are you currently under a physician's care?

If you are under a physician's care for *any* medical reason, ask your doctor if your medication or treatment will have an adverse effect on your skin. Discuss with your physician what can be safely used, and what skin care treatments you can safely receive. Don't take this lightly, the body has an intricate healing process, and even something seemingly superficial as manipulating or applying something topically to the skin can have adverse consequences.

Do you have any allergies?

Answering yes to this question may indicate that your skin could be on the sensitive side or sensitized. If you suffer from sinusitis or food or medical allergies, your skin is already sensitized to a certain degree. This doesn't mean that you will always have a reaction or that you will ever have a reaction to a product, but it's something to consider when purchasing a product line and checking product ingredients.

Do you have high blood pressure or diabetes? Are you HIV positive?

Certainly, any medical condition deserves to be noted. As we mentioned above, consult with your physician about your skin care concerns. Medicines for treatment of infection can often affect the skin. Read the label for possible side effects. Antibiotics, for example, can cause skin dryness, make you photosensitive (sensitive to sunlight), cause rashes or pigmentation changes. High blood pressure medication can cause rashes.

If you are diabetic, bruising occurs easily and healing is slow. So we don't want to use products that are particularly abrasive and there are certain skin care treatments (extensive extractions for example) that you'll want to avoid.

If you are HIV positive, it may be in some states that you can not receive treatment (because the esthetician is not allowed to treat you). Always take extreme care and speak with your physician about what is safely available to you.

Are you pregnant? Have you had a hysterectomy? Are you going through menopause? Are you on oral contraceptives?

These all have some hormonal issues going on that show up in the skin. Surely in pregnancy, we realize great care needs to be exercised in every thing we do. Though pregnancy is not a disease, there are changes that affect the whole body. Hyperpigmentation is very common and can manifest in some women as what is referred to as the mask of pregnancy or chloasma. Since every woman is different, every condition needs to be addressed as it arises. If you've not had acne until you were pregnant, then you will need to search for products to address the acne until after pregnancy. Realize that your body is never quite the same after bearing children, and you may not be able to use the same regimen you had before.

Hormonal therapy for menopause or because of a hysterectomy can wreck havoc on the skin. Hormones do that anyway. Some women experience a glowing complexion with no problem, and others are pulling their hair out over acne they never had before. You can expect anything from acne to excessive dryness, sensitivity, and pigmentation, or a combination of any of them. The same is true with contraceptives; it's a type of hormonal therapy, and your body reacts to these substances. Speak with your physician about what may occur. As in pregnancy, you'll have to address each condition as it occurs until your body adjusts or becomes as normal as its going to be.

Really, it's not as bad as it sounds! Be flexible, roll with the punches—you'll stress less if you do. You may never have a problem with any of this!

Do you exercise regularly?

A sluggish lifestyle produces a sluggish body. Good circulation replenishes and rejuvenates the cells, therefore assisting in a glowing complexion. Exercise keeps blood circulation up and stimulates lymph flow. The lymph vascular system is the method in which the body rids itself of unwanted material, such as wastes and bacteria, and also combats infection. It is separate from the circulatory system. There is no pump mechanism like a heart to produce flow as in the circulatory system. Movement of the body (muscle) promotes lymphatic movement. It keeps the cells well drained, detoxifies the body, and promotes healthy tissue. Exercise does the skin good!

Do you smoke?

In addition to the other obvious health issues related to smoking, it is believed that smoking may cause fine wrinkles and deplete the skin of vitamin C. It restricts oxygen to the skin, ages the skin, and produces a sallow or yellowing of the complexion.

Do you consume alcohol? Are you consuming caffeinated beverages?

The amount of alcohol and the frequency at which it is consumed has a drying effect on the skin. If you are consuming one or more alcoholic beverages a day (beer included), you are contributing to skin dryness and bodily dehydration, and not to mention racking up on calories. There are studies that indicate that a glass of wine is full of antioxidants, but why not take the supplements that have the same antioxidant provisions or no sugar added juices, and you won't have to worry about the alcoholic content!

Caffeine has the same affect. One caffeinated beverage is said to dehydrate the body by four eight-ounce cups of water. *Do the math.*

How much water do you drink daily?

This is crucial especially if you also consume alcohol or caffeinated beverages. (read previous paragraphs again if you've forgotten). Water is essential for survival. It is the most abundant substance in the body and present in every tissue to some degree. The blood itself is about 92 percent water, muscles about 75 percent, and bones approximately 25 percent water. Water helps to eliminate waste from the body. The body does not store water.

Side Note: Somewhere, there is a lady retaining water and is vehemently disagreeing right now, but normally the body does not retain water.

Because you have to have water in order for the body to function properly, the recommended estimated daily amount of water consumption is somewhere around at least six to eight eight-ounce glasses, depending on your body weight. This would put you at about thirty-six to forty-eight ounces of water daily on the low side. If you drink one caffeinated beverage—remember, they dehydrate the body by four cups/glasses of water—you've depleted the body of thirty-two ounces of water. If that's all you are consuming, you just wiped out much of your minimum daily requirement. Your body isn't getting enough. Your skin certainly isn't. The result can be dry, dehydrated skin and constipation—let's be real—no getting rid of wastes and toxins. What do you expect?

Do you take vitamins? Are you dieting?

Vitamins are great for the skin and for the body as a whole as long as they are taken as directed. Unless you're taking vitamins prescribed by a doctor with special instructions, please follow the recommended dosage on the labeling. If you're noticing any changes in your skin other than something good, you may want to consult a doctor.

Dieting. Dieting should be conducted with professional advice and a lot of common sense. Your body has to have some things in order to function properly. Diets that are extremely low in fats can cause skin dryness among other problems. Those that are very restrictive can seriously affect normal bodily functions and cause possible breakouts. Proceed with caution when dieting. Try to find a well-balanced deal. Seek out the help of a nutritionist or dietician to make your meal choices. A well-balanced diet produces normal body function and a healthy skin. If you don't have access to a nutritionist or dietician, eat in moderation. Try portion control by cutting back on what you normally consume, and stay away from high-calorie foods. Also, try eating six smaller meals a day instead of three large ones. Exercising makes a big difference.

How often do you experience breakouts? Are your breakouts in the form of blackheads/whiteheads? Are you being treated for acne? How about excessive oiliness?

If your breakout is limited to certain times of the month, you can more than likely attribute it to hormonal changes going on at that time. You probably do not suffer from acne if that is the only time you experience it. Stress can also produce breakout in certain areas. It is a good idea to monitor your patterns of breakout. This will help you determine what might be causing it and how best to deal with it.

Blackheads and whiteheads, the names being indicative of their appearance, are forms of congestion or buildup within a follicle. Both should be extracted (removed or cleansed) by a professional esthetician or dermatologists. Translation, don't pick your face! You want to be sure not to use products that contribute to clogging and congesting the skin. Cleanse well. Thoroughly remove makeup before retiring every night. Take care to protect the face when spraying hair care products or applying treatments to the hair.

If you are under a physician's care and using a prescription drug to address your acne concerns, if they haven't already given you a full skin care regimen (some dermatologists have estheticians on staff), ask them to refer you to an esthetician for a professional line that can work in conjunction with your medication. Also, understand the effects of the medication. Benzoyl peroxide is often found in acne prescriptions. It is known to increase photosensitivity (sensitivity to sunlight). It can also cause dryness and sensitivity.

Do you experience dryness, redness, or tightness? Do you notice any redness occurring from heat, cold, or wind exposure? Does your skin itch and burn and become easily irritated and inflamed?

If you answered yes to any or all of these types of symptoms, you may be environmentally sensitized or have sensitive skin. You want to be careful what products are applied and be sure that they don't contain known irritants. Monitor how your skin responds or reacts to a particular product, the weather, food, medicine, or even clothing.

Do you use sunscreen?

Hopefully, you answered yes. Everyone, let me repeat, everyone needs to use sunscreen or sunblock (more on these later). Choose those from a professional line if you can, they are usually less greasy than over-the-counter brands, noncomedogenic, and do not contain some of the irritants associated with UV protective ingredients.

Are you using any of the following?

- *Cleanser—Essential.* Needed to properly cleanse dirt, oils, makeup, and debris from the skin surface. Cleanser is not like regular soap.

- *Toner—Good to have.* Assists with hydrating the skin.

- *Moisturizer—Essential.* Needed to lock in moisture and protect the skin. Yes, even oily skin.

- *Exfoliant—Good to have.* Used once weekly, assists with removal of dead cellular buildup. Rejuvenates cells and stimulates cellular renewal. Keeps complexion bright.

- *Mask—Good to have.* Conditions the skin by addressing oiliness, dryness, dehydration, or premature aging, etc. Rejuvenates and replenishes cells.

- *Eye treatment cream—Good to have.* Helps to diminish the appearance of fine lines around the eyes and to protect and hydrate the eye area. Some formulations assist with decreasing puffiness and appearance of dark circles.

- *Night cream—Optional.* Formulations vary. Good for extra hydration of dry or dehydrated skin. Depends on what needs you want to address.

- *Soap and water—Better than nothing.* But they are not as effective as using a good cleanser.

- *Nothing—Not good.*

How often do you cleanse your skin?

Cleansing the face is usually part of the morning routine. Great. Cleansing the skin at night is equally important even if you don't wear makeup, but especially if you do. Cleansing is removal of everything that doesn't belong on your skin. Throughout the day, you've accumulated dirt particles, bacteria, dead skin cells, sweat, and oils. These, along with the makeup, need to be gently but effectively removed from the surface. This will ensure that your skin remains healthy. Your face may not look dirty, but it is. Proper cleansing is vital, and the success of your whole regimen is contingent on carefully executing this first step.

The questions you answered are the kinds of questions skin care therapists will ask to assist in analyzing your skin and choosing the appropriate treatments and products for you. There are different product formulations for a reason. They are there to cater to certain conditions. The more educated you are about your particular skin patterns and phases, the better you'll be prepared to address these concerns. The more information you can relay to your therapist, the better they can help you obtain your goals.

Okay, so now we know a little about what may be going on with your skin.

Our next step is to select a product that is going to address those issues and produce results. What good is it to purchase a product and use it, and after ample time it's still not working for you? What is the point of using something when it's not producing the *realistic* goals you're trying to achieve? What sense does that make?

You're armed and ready, but before you talk to an esthetician about what you want to achieve, or head to the department store with your notes and tell the woman behind the counter what you need, let's explore some things we don't want in our product line.

WHAT'S IN THE BOTTLE?

It pays to read the label. Reading is fundamental, right? There are many product lines in the market that claim one great miracle after another. All formulations are not created equal. You need to know as a consumer and as a skin savvy individual exactly what you are putting on your skin. Remember, there is no overnight cure. It took a while for your skin to become as it is, and it will take sometimes longer to get it where it should be. Practice patience and consistency.

Ingredients such as mineral oil (this is sketchy because it is said that there is cosmetic grade mineral oil—let's err, if we do, on the side of caution), petrolatum, waxes, and lanolin (ultrarefined in high-end cosmetics) can be comedogenic (cause blackheads and skin congestion) and should be avoided, especially if they are at the top of the list. These ingredients along with harsh chemicals, dyes, formaldehyde, and artificial fragrances or colors can irritate delicate skin. As much as is possible, try to steer clear of these. Check the ingredient label carefully before selecting your product line. Ask the consultant at the cosmetic counter if the product is noncomedogenic (doesn't clog the pores). If you are prone to sensitivity, check to see that there aren't any substances known to you that trigger a reaction. You don't have to become a chemist to accomplish this.

Other product items require even more care in the selection process. For instance, when looking for an exfoliant, keep in mind that gentle effective action is the key to glowing skin. Scrubs that contain large particles are too abrasive for the face and should be saved for your feet, knees, and elbows. If it hurts, it's a good indication that it's too abrasive. A formulation that uses ground particles or powder is a better choice. Excessive rubbing and massaging should be avoided. The particles work of themselves, by virtue of what they are, micro-abrasives and only light pressure should be used. Mild organic enzymatic exfoliants are wonderful. These can be a crème or mask formula (they don't usually contain particles but some may). Some ingredients you may see in these exfoliants are papaya, banana, or pumpkin. Plant derived enzymes dissolve dead cell matter without abrasive maneuvers. A sample should be obtained first or a sensitivity test performed, if at all possible, for more sensitive skin.

Skin brighteners are another product item that needs to be selected with extreme care. For skin of color, major areas of concern are an uneven complexion and dark spots. Bleaching creams are a popular choice for combating discoloration. Many over-the-counter products contain hydroquinone that blocks the action of the formation of melanin. This agent is very effective and approved by the FDA in certain strengths; however, there are some health concerns associated with it. Most professional lines (products available only through a licensed skin care center, spa/medispa or physician's office) offer an alternative to bleaching agents and are using more natural plant essences and oils in their formulations to help brighten the complexion. These natural brighteners such as mulberry and licorice have proven to be very effective. Formulations sooth and calm, help maintain oil and moisture, balance, brighten, even out the skin tone, and are natural alternatives to their chemical counterparts.

- Patience and consistency (you've seen these words before) are key objectives when using any brightening treatment.
- Time + consistency + protection = results.

Professional lines are naturally going to cost more than your drugstore varieties. High-quality active ingredients are used to effectively bring about results and are therefore more costly. Typically, drugstore versions will have lesser amounts of active ingredients or may use less effective ingredients. You'll notice the difference between the professional and drugstore brands. Granted, some people say they do fine with their drugstore varieties and are pleased. One over-the-counter brand may work better than another, but their efficacy usually does not outweigh those of professional standards. That's just a slim few out of a myriad of products available in any given line.

If you've received a professional treatment, the esthetician will recommend formulations for you to use. If you are skeptical about purchasing the full-sized product, ask if there are samples available that you can try and get enough for at least a week's worth of usage. It may be that you can purchase a travel size. This way, you're still spending less money upfront, and you can use the product for a few weeks. Most centers are more than happy to accommodate you. They would rather let you try out the product, be pleased, and return to purchase some. Keep in mind that you are making an investment in yourself. If after you've done this trial and used the samples, and your skin has done nothing but improve, there are no signs of irritation or reaction, then by all means, get the full-sized version and continue your regimen. Something else to keep in mind is that samples may not be available in every product line. In that case, you'll have to take the plunge. Please respect the profession and do not ask for samples weeks at a time to keep from purchasing the product.

Understandably, if you can not afford to go that route, do the best that you can do for right now. Don't fret. You're more skin savvy now and can compare intelligently. You can select the brand that will work for you for now and gradually work up to the more professional brands, if you desire. Our goal is to get you doing something and to keep you consistent with it. We want gentle, soothing, effective, and results-oriented products. You must keep in mind that you are a valuable asset and worthy of the best treatment possible. This is not a vanity trip. It's all about taking care of the "me" person. We do so much to care for others, it's time, and it's okay to take time out for ourselves. Another important factor to remember here is time. After you've selected a product, give the stuff time to work! Your condition did not develop overnight, and you need to give the treatment an adequate amount of time to work. You should see some clarity within the first week or two. If after at least six weeks you don't see any signs of improvement, then seek professional help or reevaluate why you chose the brand you're using.

Don't forget to check your makeup and sun care products for pore-clogging ingredients too! Often times these pore-clogging ingredients are in our foundations and such and work negatively against what we are trying to achieve.

Take care to scrutinize your body care formulations (i.e., body lotions, creams, shower gels). Cover everything that covers you!

Petroleum Jelly and Alcohol

Okay, I know I'm going to hurt someone's feelings here, but that is not my intent. There are those of you that would swear by straight petroleum jelly and alcohol. Petroleum jelly, no matter what the brand, clogs your pores! End of story. Sure, it's great for dissolving makeup and mascara, but it tends to leave a residue on your skin which will eventually accumulate in your pores and cause congestions and breakouts. Most types of waxy or thick greasy substances that aren't water-soluble substances will do the same thing. Your skin may feel smooth and hydrated (could it be the light film of grease) because the jelly does seal in moisture and prevents moisture loss, but there are better noncomedogenic formulations to use. Keep the jelly on your feet if you want to, you can even put it on your hands and use the little cotton gloves at night, but don't use it on your face.

All right, alcohol. Do we even have to go there? Too strong for anybody. End of that story. Alcohol, specifically rubbing alcohol, is too drying. It will overstrip the skin of good natural oils and exacerbate any case of acne. However, you can get in the Internet and find ten or more sites confirming your own personal beliefs. Ever notice how white or ashen the skin becomes after you have rubbed it with alcohol? Or the extremely tight feeling you get? Dryness—there you go. Astringents (often confused with toners) are notorious for containing SD alcohol (denatured alcohol); they are too drying and SD alcohol is a known skin irritant. Do not confuse plant-derived alcohols that are beneficial for conditioning the skin with the others. Look for these ingredients in your product before you buy: ethyl alcohol, methanol, benzyl alcohol, isopropyl alcohol. If any of these are at the top of the list, try to avoid the product altogether. Not an all-inclusive list, but a good place to begin. Your skin should never feel like it might crack if you blink after using any product. From a professional standpoint, there are other choices that are very effective and less harsh. The purpose of this book is to help you make better, more educated choices.

Major cosmetic manufacturers are going with all-natural formulas or those that use more plant-derived substances. They're worth checking into. Many resources are available to research product lines. Many companies are showcasing their product using the Internet. Utilize it if you can. Do your homework before you buy. Get the best that you possibly can and what works for *you*! Doing your research will pay off in the end.

Be selective. You're worth it. Go through your beautifying product assortment. Toss any and everything that contains these ingredients. Your first and most important priority is your skin. You're not in competition with your girlfriends. I know what you're thinking, "I just spent all that money on this product and makeup. I haven't even used it all!" Well, aren't you glad you found out that there was something better for you before you made things worse?

There are, as discussed earlier, plant derivatives that produce the desired results without the harshness attributed to other manufactured ingredients.

Below is a list of just a few natural ingredients that have wonderful conditioning benefits when included in skin care formulations:

- *Any skin condition.* Lavender, cucumber, chamomile, comfrey (allantoin), calendula, and aloe: soothing, calming, and healing properties.

- *Acneic/oily.* Rosemary, tea tree oil, lemon or lemongrass, echinacea, eucalyptus, witch hazel (diluted): astringent, antifungal, anti-inflammatory, and antiseptic properties.

- *Dry/dehydrated/mature.* Cucumber, vitamin E, marsh mallow, borage, hyaluronic acid (binds moisture to the skin), rich emollients such as avocado oil, jojoba oil, grapeseed oil: lubricating and conditioning emphasis properties.

- *Vitamins A, C, and E.* Antioxidants that help fight free radicals. Vitamin K and the properties in blueberries help fight pigmentation issues.

To do:

1. Study skin and decide which condition closely describes present experience with skin. Decide on a condition. Seek help/confirmation from therapist. Log it in your skin care journal.

2. Research product brands. Look for natural ingredients and absence of harsh substances and

those that are non-comedogenic. Write the products you select in your journal.

3. Speak with consultant or set up skin analysis with esthetician.

4. After trial period, purchase product if favorable improvement noticed in skin. Write the names of the product that will become part of your regimen in your journal.

5. Remain focused, and be consistent in regimen to obtain skin care goals.

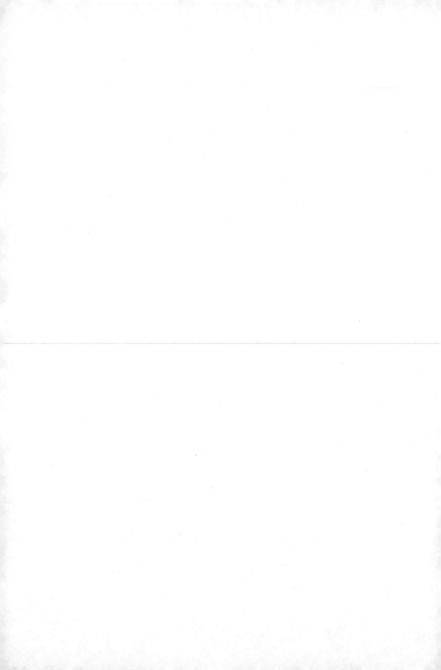

SKIN FITNESS—A WORKOUT REGIMEN

Every year, millions of us start out the New Year with resolutions and good intentions to change our lives for the better, only to get frustrated, worn out, or suffer from temporary Alzheimer's (forgetting all about our pledges) after six weeks.

Hey, it needn't be that way, especially when it comes to taking care of our skin. With skin care, it is important to be consistent—true—but there's an easy way to make a lifelong commitment to maintain healthy skin. Skin fitness is a very achievable goal for every man, woman, and child. In as little as ten to fifteen minutes a day total (five minutes in the morning and five minutes at night—maybe ten if you wear makeup) and twenty minutes extra once or twice a week, you'll take your skin's fitness level to new heights (or brights!). Your outer covering will be in tip-top shape in no time. How, you ask? I'll show you.

Let's begin a skin fit exercise assuming you've very carefully selected the best product you can suited to your budget, and one you know you'll be committed to using.

Every morning when you arise, you (hopefully) make your way to the bathroom to clean your face, brush your teeth, etc., and perform all of your other grooming habits. Well, here's a routine that fits right in with your morning ritual.

To get started, first, brush your teeth. Wet your washcloth in warm water. Clean that good night's rest out of your eyes! Apply your cleanser (you should only have to use a small amount) to damp hands and using fingertips massage over the face and neck with light upward rotating strokes for approximately one minute. Rinse. If you slept with your makeup on, apply cleanser again. Massage. Rinse. Apply hydration (moisturizer) while skin is still damp with toner. Apply solar protection.

Voila! You're all set! That's it.

It can't be that easy, you say? But it is.

The first part of any good regimen is adequately cleaning the skin. Got it? Good.

1. Massage the cleanser for approximately a minute to ensure that all dirt and dead cell buildup has been adequately removed. Rinse well.

2. Lightly apply toner, then while the skin is damp, quickly apply moisturizer immediately after toning to lock in moisture.

3. Apply solar protection to protect against UV damage.

Five to seven minutes tops—every morning. It can't get any easier than this.

Apply your makeup, do your hair, get dressed, etc., and carry on having a wonderfully blessed day. If you shower in the morning, you can apply your cleanser in the shower. Same process: apply, massage, and rinse. Good. Upon exiting the shower, blot excess water and sprits your face with the toner, follow with hydration and protection.

At night, you especially want to repeat the process to thoroughly remove makeup and the oils and dust that have gathered on your skin throughout the day. Start by removing your eye makeup. Mascara can take a little extra time, so begin with this first. Let your cleanser set on the eye area for about twenty seconds (eyes closed of course) to dissolve and breakdown the makeup. (If you don't have a cleanser gentle enough for this area, use a gentle eye makeup remover instead.) Allowing the cleanser to sit will keep you from rubbing excessively around the delicate eye area; of course, you want to be sure to keep the cleanser out of the eyes. Massage the rest of the cleanser on the other areas while you leave the eye area for last. You don't have to see, you can feel the areas of your face. Gently massage the eye area with light strokes. Use soft cotton, cotton swabs, or a warm washcloth to facilitate removal of mascara. Rinse face thoroughly, cupping the hands over the eyes and bathing the face in tepid water. Be sure to remove all traces of cleanser from around the hairline.

Apply second cleansing if necessary. Rinse. Tone. Hydrate. Special therapy (i.e., night creams, eye treatments, etc.).

Taking It to Another Level Once or Twice a Week

Once (normal/dry/mature/sensitive skin) to twice (oily/acne prone skin) a week, exfoliate and/or apply a mask.

So you're saying, "I thought this was a quick thing?" It still is, so understand what we do and why, and let's do it right. Okay, so how do we exfoliate and stay within our five-minute range?

Because exfoliation is something you only need to do one time in any given day once, and usually only once a week, you can choose to do it in the morning or evening. Here's a shortcut: instead of cleansing, exfoliating, toning, etc., you're going to take your cleansing to another level. This process combines cleansing and exfoliating into one step. If you have a physical exfoliant, one containing small particles to loosen dead cells, combine a small amount of this with your cleanser to save steps. If you have an enzymatic exfoliant or one that requires that you leave it on for a little while, do something else while you're waiting. Iron your clothes, put on your hose, or select your outfit for the day if you haven't already. You're allowed to multitask! You can save it for your evening workout if you prefer.

After the first cleansing (if removing previous day's makeup—a habit you are quickly learning to break), with hands dampened, pour a small amount of cleanser and exfoliant into palm. Rub hands together to mix the two. Gently massage the face for one minute. Do not apply extra pressure. The exfoliant works under its own power. Avoid the eye area, but pay close attention to chin and forehead, especially if you are prone to breakout. Gently massage on the lobes of and around the nostrils, an area where there is frequent dead cell buildup and excess oil; use extreme care as this area is also prone to sensitivity.

Rinse well. Follow with toning and hydration.

Exfoliating is a great way to smooth the skin surface and to help even out the skin tone.

Exfoliation removes dead skin cells, stimulates circulation for healthy nourishment to the cells, and promotes cellular growth. Exfoliating gives your skin a youthful glow. Caution: too much of a good thing can be counterproductive. Be careful to never overexfoliate. This contributes to sensitizing the skin. The purpose is to gently remove the cells to maintain a healthy glow. Dead cells discolor the skin and can make darker skin appear dull and ashen. Unless you have a specially formulated exfoliant with instructions to use more often, or a condition that might dictate a different regimen (i.e. oily and sometimes hyperpigmented skin) stick to the once a week program.

Let's move on to the mask. The mask can serve many purposes depending upon the formulation. Some masks are for hydrating (cream or gel), some for drawing out debris and absorbing oils (clay), and tightening or refining (creamy with some clay properties). Some are allowed to dry and others are not. Some are removed by peeling them off, others rubbed or rinsed off.

Every product is selected according to your skin's needs so choosing your mask is going to be no different. Be sure to check the formulations and find one suitable to address your needs.

- Clay masks are great for oilier skin as they absorb excess oil and help draw out impurities and buildup.

- Medicated masks are also available. They're great acne fighters.

- Gel masks can be for hydrating, purifying, or refining. Look for a hydrating base for dry/dehydrated skin. Another suitable choice would be a cream-based hydrating mask. Purifying is more for acne or blemish-prone skin, and refining mask for mature or sun-damaged skin. Read each label carefully because sometimes terminology for one company can be totally different from another, so refining for one may be for blemishes and to others, for working on mature devitalized skin. I know, go figure? But it happens.

- For combination skin, you may end up buying two masks—one to hydrate the drier areas and one to apply to the oily areas. Do whatever works.

Adapt your way of thinking and overcome obstacles (complaining about having to buy two or use two) by your actions (working to reach the skin care goals you've set for yourself).

If you are unsure as to what to use, remember you can always seek the advice of a qualified esthetician.

Whether you mask in the morning or evening is up to you. You'll begin with your regular cleansing. Rinse. Instead of toning at this point, apply your mask. If your mask calls for setting perhaps for ten to twenty minutes, why not consider doing the mask at night? This will allow you time to relax and perhaps hydrate the rest of your body if you've just showered. Applying your mask after showering is most beneficial because the pores are dilated and the skin softened making it most receptive and responsive to the beneficial properties contained in the formula. After allowing the mask to set for the required time, rinse thoroughly. Pay close attention to the hairline, near the ears, and the jaw line. Towel dry to damp. Spritz with toner. Hydrate immediately. Voila! You're finished.

You can easily keep this skin solution for the rest of your life! So if you really look at the time involved in maintaining healthy skin, it's very minimal, the results however can be amazing.

Special Note:

Just a quick note about the importance of the steps in your skin fitness regimen. As stated earlier, your cleanser is an important first step. The toner, an often overlooked component provides extra hydration for all skin conditions. Toners are different from astringents. Astringents are drying and remove oils – toners are hydrating and moisturizing and topically add water content to the skin. Depending on its formulation it can be used not only to hydrate but for sensitive skin, for instance, it can calm and soothe; for mature skin – provide extra moisture and antioxidants; for oily skin hydration and soothing for inflamed skin; for dry skin – extra hydration and healing. If you haven't already done so, as soon as it's within your budget, add the beneficial properties of the toner to your daily regimen.

Another point that needs to be highlighted is for those suffering from oily/acneic skins that do not use a moisturizer. Regardless of whether your skin is oily you need to use a moisturizer to keep the "water" content up. Moisturizing for oily skin is targeted in reducing oil production but keeping a proper water balance to bring about a "normalized" or as close to normalized condition as possible. Do not neglect this step ever.

Finally, people of color do need to use solar protection...period. It does not matter that you don't think so. The fact still remains the damage is still taking place.

Too many times we allow hurdles to slow or block our progress in reaching our goals. Whether it's trying to lose weight and we have one more helping than needed or in working our way to a more clear complexion but utilizing ineffective products to do so. The actions in both of these scenarios slow our progress and hinder reaching our long awaited goals.

Taking time-out to cleanse, tone, hydrate, and protect your skin at all times will save you headache, heartache, and money. When you are diligent about keeping your skin in excellent condition through treatments, therapies, and premium products you're not only maintaining what you have, but you also allow for constant improvement in your skin's fitness. It's not unlike building muscle with intense training and then laying out of the gym for several weeks. When you relax your strategies, you may end up having to start all over again.

Moral of the story: maintain your steady pace—continue with maximum at home care with premium skin products and regularly-planned visits to your skin care therapist. This strategy will not only keep you in the competition, but allow you to reach your goals with confidence.

Note: There are many premium lines that incorporate botanical ingredients into their formulations but may not be considered an all-"natural" line—this is okay. Great care is utilized to present a quality effective product.

WHAT'S UP WITH THIS?

We've all had skin breakouts and other occurrences that we've never experienced before. Okay. Well, the majority of us have major or minor—it doesn't matter. Sometimes products that we've used for years suddenly produce angry inflamed skin. Life changes, hormones, pregnancy, menopause, and aging begin to take their toll on the whole body, and we don't like the changes they put us through. This chapter focuses on those cycles in our life that begin to wreck havoc on the whole of one's person. Each of the topics covered here whether alone or in combination with others has adverse affects on the skin and our own self-esteem. Learning the causes (remember our skin conditions chart in the chapter "What about Me?") and effects helps us to better deal with and manage the outcome produced by these different "traumas," boosting control of these traumas in our favor. We control them, they do not control us. Another thing to always keep in mind is that whether you like it or not, your body will change (if it didn't, you wouldn't be so concerned about trying to keep your girlish figure). That said, from time to time, you will find that you may have to and probably will need to adjust your skin care game. It's just a matter of rolling with the punches and continuing to move ahead.

How Stress Affects the Skin

First, stress is no joke. Stress is a killer. It methodically breaks down the body and weakens its systems. It can cause migraines, heart attack, and stroke. Stress is known to lead to hair loss, ulcers, heart attack, and a deficient immune system. This is bad enough, and we haven't even started on what it can do to the skin!

Have you noticed the increasing number of TV ads for new drugs on the market? These ads feature drugs to treat everything that ails you—allergies, intimacy problems, depression, and there's even drugs to help you handle stress!

Wow! What a scary thought to realize that so many treatments for what ails you are in a bottle. Not to mention the whole slew of side affects that go along with them.

Stress is a very real and very serious problem. It affects the body both physically and psychologically. No matter what color the skin, stress in any form is bad.

Although equipped to handle stressful situations, the Lord did not intend that the body remain in a stress reactive mode.

So what is stress?

Acute stress, or short-term stress, commonly referred to as "fight or flight" response is a mechanism God put into humans to help us react quickly to a threatening situation.

When an individual encounters a threat, the body kicks into overdrive to be ready to respond to the threat; either to fight or to turn and flee. There are many hormones released during a stressful episode. Interestingly enough, the heart rate and blood pressure increase instantaneously. Breathing becomes rapid as the lungs take in more oxygen. Blood flow can increase dramatically readying the muscles, lungs, and brain for added demands and is diverted away from skin (producing cool, clammy, and sweaty skin). The spleen releases red and white cells allowing the blood to transport more oxygen. Systems that are not needed are shutdown temporarily as well as nonessential body functions. Fluids are diverted from the mouth causing dryness and difficulty in talking. Spasms can begin in the throat, making it difficult to swallow. Recognize any of these? When was the last time you were scared?

Once all threat of harm has passed, and there have been no harmful effects, the stress hormone level returns to normal. The relaxation response sets in as your body systems also normalize. Acute stress is good as it protects one from harm.

On the flip side is chronic stress. Unfortunately, everyday life can pose on-going stressful situations that are not short term, and thus the urge to act (fight or flight) must be suppressed. Stress then becomes chronic. Long-term relationship problems, on-going high-pressured job situations, financial worries, peer pressure, fear and anxiety are just a few common chronic stressors. An accumulation of persistent stressful situations, particularly those that a person cannot easily control, a traumatic event, or the inability of the body to produce sufficient relaxation response, are most likely to produce negative physical effects. There are studies that suggest that a person's inability to adapt to stress is associated with the onset of depression or anxiety. Evidence suggests that stress diminishes the quality of life by reducing feelings of pleasure and accomplishment. Other studies link stress to hypertension, stroke, susceptibility to infections, irritable bowel syndrome, insulin resistance (diabetes), tension headaches, muscular and joint pain, and sleep disturbances.

Let's buy a clue. If we know that stress does all of those things to the inside of the body, would it be safe to assume that it certainly isn't helping the outside either?

Some of the first signs of stress will be evident in the paleness of the skin (lack of proper diet practices), dark circles under the eyes (insomnia), wrinkles, and lines from furrowing the brows (worrying about those "threatening" situations), just to name a few. According to one study, how an individual reacts to stress influences how easily they resist or succumb to a disease (remember, the skin is the first line of defense against disease). They came to the conclusion that "introverts" are less able to fight illness than extroverts because they release more of the stress hormone! Remember the fearsome different hormones produced in the body when a person is under stress? Cortisol and testosterone are two of them. Cortisol produces pigmentation and is believed to be connected to weight gain in women, and testosterone can cause acneic breakout and hair growth! Not where you want it. *Like we need that.* Not very becoming in females. Skin conditions such as hives, acne, rosacea, eczema, and psoriasis are believed to be caused and/or exacerbated by stress.

Ladies, look, why do we go through the process of doing the hair, nails, and skin, only to look like a washout because we let people and circumstances get on our nerves? Have you ever heard anyone say, "They're about to worry me to death?" Hello! They can and will if you allow it. Calm nerves, adequate rest, and of course, excellent skin care will keep us looking vibrant, not embalmed!

What do we do about stress? How do we combat the affects of stress? Well, one of the first things we want to do is to have our quiet time with the Lord. Meditate on these verses of the Scripture. This beats any and all stress control therapies.

> Great peace have they which love thy law: and nothing shall offend them.
>
> Psalms 119:165 (KJV)

> Thou wilt keep him in perfect peace whose mind is stayed on thee: because he trusteth in thee.
>
> Isaiah 26:3

I will lift up mine eyes unto the hills, from whence cometh my help. My help cometh from the Lord, which made heaven and earth. He will not suffer thy foot to be moved: he that keepeth thee will not slumber. Behold, he that keepeth Israel shall neither slumber nor sleep. The Lord is thy keeper: the Lord is thy shade upon thy right hand. The sun shall not smite thee by day, nor the moon by night. The Lord shall preserve thee from all evil: he shall preserve thy soul. The Lord shall preserve thy going out and thy coming in from this time forth, and even for evermore.

Psalms 121

In other words—know Jesus, no stress; no Jesus, know stress! This is for you. Substitute your name for personal pronouns whenever possible. Make it personal because it is. Stress kills and destroys inside and out. Don't let it have the victory over you. Write in your journal at the back of the book all the things that stress you throughout the day on a regular basis or whatever. Think about each one. Are these things that you can personally do something about? Do you need to settle issues with others? Make a commitment to yourself to not let stress have the rule over your life.

After you have your quiet time, the second thing you need to concentrate on is breaking out of the stress cycle. This is the routine you allow yourself to go through day in and day out, whether on the job or at home. Break out! Do something different. Don't let people and situations cause you to become reactive. Remain calm, pray, don't head for the fridge, don't beat your desk (or your boss), and please don't pick blemishes! Find ways to turn things around. Take on the *customer service* mentality—ask your coworker, boss, spouse, or kids what you can do to help alleviate any problems. Perhaps they don't realize there is one, and you have to bring it to their attention. Be proactive. When you decide to be proactive instead of reactive, you are in control of the situation. Frustration and pent up emotions which have been suppressed can come into play in a positive way and bring about closure to stress-related issues. The realization that this is part of taking care of yourself and good for your personal well-being should be motivation enough to pursue resolution. Being proactive in stress reduction increases and boosts your self-esteem. Who doesn't feel good about confronting issues head-on and taking charge of one's life?

Third (this is clearly one of the best parts of the whole therapy), take a time out for you!

Here are suggestions for some quality *me* time.

Head for the spa! Your skin care therapist is a great resource for stress-relieving treatments. Some services involve the use of aromatherapy and relaxing music to soothe and calm the muscles and nerves, and you can combat those wrinkles while you're at it! A facial massage is excellent for relieving tension in facial muscles and relief from headaches (sinusitis included). Check out your local spa and see what they have to offer.

Can't make it to the spa? Create your own spa atmosphere at home. Begin with scented candles or fragrant melting wax or aromatic sprays. Take a warm shower with your favorite bath gel (one free from all irritating ingredients) or soak in the tub using bath oil, Dead Sea mineral salts, or Epsom salts with an essential oil blend added for fragrance and effect. The fragrance will scent the whole room. If you just want to lie on the bed after a long day, or candles are not available, fill your bathroom sink with a little warm water and pour your gel/oil in for a nice pleasant aroma. Add some ambience with soothing instrumental music. (Singing is nice but sometimes hard to relax to.) There are some excellent instrumental gospel CDs available that promote peace, praise, and relaxation.

Grab a nice warm cup of decaf tea (a good herbal blend that is loaded with antioxidants) and a good book (our favorite is the Bible) relax, and read for a while. There are many specialty tea stores that offer superb tea blends for your enjoyment.

Wash your hair and use an herbal infusion of lavender as a final rinse (take about ten ounces of dried herbs or a large handful of fresh herbs and boil in two and a half cups of water for about ten minutes. Strain and allow cooling to a comfortable temperature). It smells *so* good and will help you feel relaxed. Sit under the dryer with your decaf tea and book! *Do not do this if you are pregnant or suspect that you are, or if you are breastfeeding.*

Use the same infusion and pour it in bathwater. *Do not do this if you are pregnant or suspect that you are, or if you are breastfeeding.*

Essential oils may also be added to a bath. Sprinkle five to ten drops in water that is warm, but not hot. Don't add them under hot running water as they will evaporate and you'll lose the therapeutic benefits. If your skin is dry, add the oils in a tablespoon of almond oil (*not if you're allergic to nuts!*). Some good choices again are chamomile, lavender, and jasmine. Aromatherapy blends are also available and have general names or descriptions such as "relaxing" blend or "rejuvenating" blend or something of that nature. Choose your blends from a reputable source. Use extreme caution when using essential oils. They are very, very potent. Better yet, go to the store or spa and buy a blend such as those mentioned above to add to your bathwater. *Do not do this if you are pregnant or suspect that you are, or if you are breastfeeding.*

There is a message here. So pay attention.

When at the office, use your breaks! If you have a fifteen-minute break, go for a short walk (as long as you can do it in safety). If seating is available outside your place of work, grab your book and sit under the trees for a while. If you have your own office—close and lock the door, turn off the lights (you can leave the desk light on), shut your eyes. The possibilities are endless. If you get two breaks throughout the day, so much the better, just don't take them both at the same time.

Bring your relaxing CDs to work and play them on low in your office, upload them to your MP3 player or phone, and listen to them while on break.

The important thing to remember is to have a channel to get rid of stress. No one wants to look years older than they really are. Don't let stress rob you of your youth!

On another note, well, not entirely, but anyway, ladies, we are typically the hub of the family. If we're stressed out, the whole family knows it, and our family feels our stress. Let's bring peace to our homes by handling this issue and stopping the ripple effect in our homes. Amen.

Acne

Acne can be a most debilitating skin condition robbing persons of their self-esteem and contributing to depression and anxiety in many individuals. It's no wonder that when we surveyed one hundred black women about skin concerns, acne ranked number two as a major problem (hyperpigmentation was number one).

Acne affects the sebaceous follicles and hair follicles of the skin. It is a genetic disease that causes the malfunction of the pilosebaceous unit. This unit consists of the hair shaft; sebaceous gland, which makes the sebum (oil); the erector pili muscle, which makes hair stand on end when contracted; and the hair follicle. The trouble begins when dead skin cells are shed at an abnormally high rate; compounding this development is the release of the sebum of oily skin that is thicker than normal. This combination of a rapid production of dead cells along with thick sebum contributes to clogging of pores and a lack of oxygen in the follicles. This is a perfect environment for the *Propionibacterium acnes* (P acnes, a.k.a. acne bacteria) which naturally resides in the follicles to multiply. These bacteria react with the sebum and produce waste products that irritate the lining of the follicle and cause inflammation, producing pain, pustules and blemishes, and ultimately... low self-esteem.

As with any skin condition, it takes time to heal or bring about a balance to acneic skin. Be patient. Even with clinical care, clearing will not take place overnight and should not be expected to. In the medical and esthetic industry, acne is divided into four grades of severity. Number one is mild—common among teens. Grade 2 (inflammation/pustules) is usually associated with comedogenic cosmetic ingredients or poor and improper cleansing habits. There are some pustules and inflammation. Grade 3 (excessive pustules/inflammation) is due to an imbalance of hormones and should be treated by a dermatologist. There are excessive pustules and inflammation in this stage. Grade 4 is cystic acne with characteristics of nodules, cysts, and pustules and should be treated by a dermatologist.

There are the many things that can trigger acne flare-ups:

- *Stress.* We discussed that earlier, but for review purposes, stress causes the stimulation of testosterone (in women) which results in an unnatural increase in the production of sebum (oil).

- *Hormones.* Fluctuations at certain times of the month, contraceptive pills, and menopause can contribute to breakout depending on whether there is an increase in androgens (testosterone) or estrogen.

- *Heat and humidity.* These increase oil production and blood flow, and cause you to sweat providing a breeding ground for bacteria.

- *Cosmetics.* Ingredients in cosmetics can clog pores and cause irritation to hair follicles.

- *Friction.* The rubbing or constant moving of something against the skin can cause trauma and stimulate oil flow.

One of the best ways to begin fighting acne is to try to remove the triggers associated with it. Practice some of the stress relief methods in the previous subchapter. It's an inexpensive way to fight breakout! Second, address the condition by using proper cleansing products and procedures to cleanse without stripping, combat oil production, fight infection and bacteria, and promote healing. As discussed in the chapter "What's in the Bottle?" check your product label and know what you're using. Too many times, people have selected products that are too harsh and end up worsening their acneic condition. Anything that strips your skin to the point that it's now excessively dry and tight will only cause the sebaceous glands to produce *more* oil. Washing the face too often (refer to the chapter Skin Fitness for proper cleansing methods) can overdry the skin prompting it to produce more oil also. Know what you need or at least have an idea; this is why a customized skin care regimen is important (refer to "Why Customized Skin Care Is Important"). We're looking for products that heal, sooth, calm, are clearing, and antibacterial. At the end of the chapter "What's in the Bottle?" we listed some ingredients that are very helpful in combating acne.

Special Note: A few blemishes before and during that time of month do not an acneic skin make!

Seeking the advice and care of an esthetician will help you achieve the reachable goal of clear, blemish-free skin. When you visit the esthetician, she/he will thoroughly analyze and cleanse your skin and probably perform a procedure called extracting, a method in which an extractor, or sometimes, the esthetician's skilled fingers are used to work debris out of the skin, thereby cleansing the pores. A disincrustation fluid may be applied under vapor steaming to soften the skin and to expedite removal of debris. The esthetician is specially trained to use this technique to remove blackheads and to relieve skin congestion. Acne lesions should not be picked or squeezed as this will traumatize the skin and can cause scarring and hyperpigmentation. So don't pick at your blemishes! Another benefit of going to the skin care center for treatment is the availability of soothing and calming treatments that have antibacterial properties and a healing nature. Consistent visits to your skin care provider coupled with a good home care regimen will help to combat the effects of acne and help to clear the skin. Sometimes you may have to purchase extra products to work with your cleanser and moisturizer. These may be a spot treatment with benzoyl peroxide or natural salicylic acid, an oil control solution, or something to help calm inflammation. Product lines have varied treatment modalities.

Another thing to do is to check your diet. Are you drinking enough water? Water is essential in keeping the body flushed of toxins. Have you begun a rigorous exercise regimen? Sweat and bacteria or use of a soiled towel can contribute to breakout. Make sure you cleanse your skin well after exercising. Do not be tempted, however, to overwash the skin; instead, make sure you are using the correct products to help control oil production. Overwashing stimulates the oil glands, and that's not what you're trying to do! As mentioned in the chapter "Your Customized Skin Care," it is a good idea to monitor breakout or any changes. This can be as simple as jotting the word "breakout" on your calendar and perhaps where it is occurring. You'll have something you can reference and an easy way to notice if you were going through cycles of stress, hormones, climatic changes, increased physical activity, etc. Be sure to change and launder your pillowslips on a regular basis, as natural and hair product oils, dead skin, and dirt tends to build up on the surface. If you are serious about combating acne, the time you put into this should be viewed as you're making a sound investment in yourself and it's definitely worth the extra effort to log these occurrences.

Sensitive versus Sensitized Skin— There's a Difference

You may have said it before, "Oh, my skin is so sensitive." This is a common remark that esthetician's hear on a daily basis. Is your skin really sensitive? Perhaps you may be what we in the industry call—sensitized. How can you know the difference?

Many people believe that they have sensitive skin. Do you break out after the application of some cream or lotion? How long after the application do you experience the irritation? Perhaps you can no longer use fragrances or perfumed products. Do you experience itching, burning, or inflammation? Are you prone to redness, turning red in extremes of temperature whether cold or hot? Do you flush easily? Are you fair-skinned?

Your responses to these questions have a lot to do with determining whether you're "sensitive" or "sensitized."

What is sensitive skin?

Sensitive skin is usually a characteristic (but not limited to) of fair-complexioned persons. These individuals flush easily, are prone to redness in cool and warm weather. Their skin is easily agitated by things they come into contact with (i.e., detergents, plants, dyes in clothing, environment, etc.), and typically develop a rash or redness and inflammation immediately after coming in contact with the irritant. Artificial fragrances and dyes are annoying as the skin reacts to most anything. Sensitive skin burns easily even on cloudy days and has to be thoroughly protected with a physical sunblock. Often, there is a family history of allergies of some sort, and it is believed that sensitivity may be inherited. The individual is already considered to be in a supersensitive position. Allergies to food, dust, or pollen means there are already histamines present in the body. *(When histamines are present, the immune system is being stimulated, that's why antihistamines are used to treat allergic reaction.)*

After looking at these factors, we've probably eliminated half of you that thought you had sensitive skin.

What is sensitized skin?

Unlike sensitive skin, sensitized skin seems to have no genetic connection. Environmental factors and your personal space play a large part in the causes of this condition. Reaction to a substance may take hours, days, even a number of years. The symptoms experienced by both the sensitive and sensitized may be similar—such as itching or stinging, but the sensitized skin usually will not react immediately. It really takes a little homework to find out which side a person tends to lean to. Do you see how journaling breakout and other occurrences can help you pinpoint possible triggers? Take a second to jot it on your calendar or put it on your PDA, phone, tablet, or whatever, so you'll have a reference to refer back to.

This Never Bothered Me Before

Ever wonder why you could use a product for years, and all of a sudden you begin to have breakouts and irritation for no apparent reason? It's your favorite soap or makeup, it never bothered you before, so why now?

Your skin has gradually become sensitized to that product or to the ingredients contained therein. As we discussed in earlier chapters, ingredients in our skin care products and cosmetics can promote irritation. This is why we shop for irritant-free products as much as possible.

It works like this. The body has a defense mechanism of specialized cells that work to provide protection against an invading irritant. Most of the time, these cells can surround the irritant and absorb it before it does any harm to the system or before it stimulates the immune system into action. As we age, these cells begin to decrease (I know, just one more thing to add to the aging list). Sun exposure also kills off a great many of these cells. As the body has fewer sentries now, the "enemy" is able to slip in. So where there once was peace, you now feel the effects of a battle (i.e., itching, inflammation, etc.) as your body fights against the invading substance. You begin to see evidence in the form of red itchy blotches or breakout. It is a localized reaction— limited to the application area or areas.

Some skin disorders associated with sensitivities include different forms of dermatitis. You've probably heard of different forms of dermatitis. A reaction from a piece of jewelry that contains nickel is a form of dermatitis, so is coming in contact with poison ivy.

Other causes of inflammation and/or irritation can be attributed to acts performed by the individual such as using too much of a good thing. You know what I'm talking about here. You've purchased a product, used it once or twice. The skin is looking great. You say to yourself, "Hey, if I use this three times a week instead of once a week, I'll see results faster!" Not! Lack of proper skin care and abuse of the skin by using too much of a product more than recommended can damage or impair the natural barrier function. Over-exfoliating, for example is detrimental to the health of the skin. Exfoliating excessively or more than recommended leaves the skin raw and vulnerable to attack.

When addressing sensitivity, we still come full circle to the standards set in the chapters "Why Customized Skin Care Is Important" and "What's in the Bottle?" Knowing your skin and knowing how to read a product label saves you a world of trouble. Sampling programs also allow you the privilege of using a product without buying a lot of it initially and being able to test for sensitivity without spending a lot of money.

Special Note: Please respect the industry professionals and not abuse a free sample program. If you've used it once and it works buy it and be done with it. Let's not keep going back for freebies.

Pay close attention to climatic conditions if you find you are sensitive/sensitized.

Adapting your regimen for different climatic and weather conditions is essential. Be prepared as much as possible, especially when traveling. Get your essentials together before you leave, and you'll be less likely to trigger a reaction, and do much to prevent your skin from reacting to a new environment. Don't count on finding what you need once you arrive!

Monitor your diet for possible triggers (seafood, caffeine, spicy foods, etc.) if you've been experiencing symptoms (inflammation, redness, itching, etc). Be sure to take vitamins and medication as directed.

Other culprits that may also trigger sensitivity are hormonal changes such as puberty, pregnancy, and menopause. Long-term stress can cause chemical imbalances and lead to disruption of the immune system (read more about stress and stress relievers in the chapter "What's Up with This?").

Exposure to outdoor or indoor pollution puts us under environmental assault. There is a natural supply of Vitamin E that defends membranes and lipids from ozone attack. This supply is constantly bombarded by free radicals. When it is then readily exhausted, the skin is vulnerable to sensitivity and aging. Whew!

Neglecting your covering may result in a reaction that could leave scarring or hyperpigmented areas. Taking the time to prevent a problem is easier than treating a condition after it has already occurred. Who needs the added stress ("How Stress Effects the Skin")?

It is important for you to reveal any reactions you may have had to any substance to your esthetician. This information is vital in determining exactly what can safely be used on your skin. Be alert to these triggers (the above list is not all inclusive) when shopping for skin, body, and hair care products. The more you familiarize yourself with and monitor changes in your skin, the more you will be less likely to experience a reaction. This information will also be useful to your dermatologist in determining the cause of a severe reaction.

Individuals suffering from rosacea, couperose, or other highly sensitized conditions would benefit greatly from a specialized treatment by a therapist. You can relax and enjoy these therapies that are incorporated to calm the skin, reduce redness, and inflammation associated with your problems. Your therapist can choose the right combination of products to help keep your skin under control and looking good. On your own, look for water-based products. Oil-based and heavy cream products trap heat and can trigger flare-ups. Keep your routine simple—cleanse, tone, moisturize, and protect. Remember to use sunblock. Use a light, gentle touch. Select hypoallergenic products that contain skin soothers: aloe vera, chamomile, and lavender, just to name a few.

So whether you are sensitive or sensitized, either way, proper skin care will keep you looking good, and no one will ever know except you, your doctor, or therapist.

Hyperpigmentation

For women of color, hyperpigmentation is a problem that is more than skin-deep. This condition is very often, unfortunately, a major cause of low self-esteem. Everyone dreams of a beautiful complexion with an even texture and uniform tone. There are many different causes of hyperpigmentation. Dark spots, or hyperpigmentation, are frustrating and never seem to fade away fast enough with the multitude of creams and ointments available on the market.

There is hope, however, for the distressed. Some understanding of what hyperpigmentation is will help to clarify seemingly tedious procedures for treatments performed esthetically and medically or in a combination of both.

In the chapter "What about Me?" we discussed the black don't crack theory and spoke of how melanin (melanocytes, more accurately) are distributed through the layers of skin (each layer is made up of cells). These are the cells that control or add "pigment" to the skin, thus creating the varied hues of people all across the globe. This is a really oversimplified explanation as the process is quite involved and intricate. They define your characteristic skin tone. Regardless of skin color, the number of melanocytes does not vary among humans. The amount of melanin in the skin is determined by genetics, but can be influenced by the environment (i.e., sunlight). The primary function of melanin is believed to be to protect the skin from sunlight. The melanin on the surface of the skin helps absorb UV light, protecting the cells below. People of color are genetically more resistant, but not immune, to UV damage because of the surface melanin cover. Alas, skin with more melanin tends to have more hyperpigmentation related to scarring.

When some form of aggression is asserted against the skin (i.e., sunlight, trauma), the pigment-producing cells go into overdrive to try to protect the skin against damage and typically do not return to normal production once the threat is gone. This results in hyperpigmentation as we know it. Acne scarring is a common result of this process. This is why dark spots may appear after you have "picked" at a blemish.

The sun is one of the skin's worst enemies. Pigmentation can accumulate over the years due to a lack of proper protection. Adequate sun protection is a must especially in darker skin tones.

Another culprit of unbalanced skin tone is due to hormonal imbalance. Pregnancy, birth control pills, or other hormone-influencing factors can stimulate the production of melanin.

In pregnancy, there is a condition referred to as the "mask of pregnancy." During the pregnancy, the mother may develop a discoloration on the neck or face appearing darker than the rest of the surrounding skin. The mask may fade sometime after pregnancy, or it may remain for many years. Studies indicate that three-fourths of pregnant women are affected by this condition.

Hormones in these substances, and those released while going through these bodily changes, influence these conditions greatly.

Skin that is wounded or inflamed can trigger overproduction of pigmentation. An allergic reaction to allergy-producing substances (particularly those causing a rash to develop) can cause adequate inflammation to sufficiently traumatize the skin. Usually, darker skin tones suffer from this type of discoloration more severely, and for a longer period of time.

The birthmark, another form of pigmentation, extends into the deeper layers of the skin and is usually inherited.

These are just some of the types and causes of hyperpigmentation. Let's take a look at a couple of treatments that are available to help address this condition.

Proper skin care hygiene is of great importance we know to minimize breakout and other trauma to the skin. *You've heard this throughout the whole book, must be important.* Practicing proper care will reduce our chances of scarring from breakout. The use of adequate sun protection will help to keep areas from coloring even more noticeably.

The depth of the pigmentation will determine its ability to be treated. Pigmentation from the sun is the easiest to treat. Post-inflammatory pigmentation or pigmentation due to a rash or breakout is more difficult to treat. The most difficult to treat is the hormonally induced pigmentation.

For many years, hydroquinone was considered the most effective ingredient for lightening the skin. Used in concentrations of up to 2 percent, the FDA authorized its usage as an over-the-counter topical drug. Hydroquinone is a very effective lightener; however, there is a high incidence of allergic occurrences and many reports of irritation associated with prolonged use. According to the Occupational Safety and Health Administration (OSHA), hydroquinone has cancer-causing potential.

There are other less traumatizing approaches to treating this condition. Since skin care is our focus, let's try to steer clear of anything that would cause any further trauma. Alternative methods to treat hyperpigmentation include using products containing botanical brighteners to inhibit the production of melanin. Many professional skin care companies have incorporated the use of homeopathic resources into their formulations to provide effective treatments against hyperpigmentation. Be patient; results may begin to take anywhere from eight to twelve weeks or more. Some spas may offer a "complexion" therapy of sorts. These treatments can involve visiting a skin care professional for the initial skin brightening treatment(s) and maintaining a strict regimen at home. Consult with your skin care therapist for an analysis of your skin condition to try to pinpoint the cause of the hyperpigmentation. Since no two people will respond the same way, do not measure your progress with that of another, okay?

During receiving and after completing any type of treatment designed to even the skin tone and involving the topical application of product(s) and/or advanced therapies (i.e., microdermabrasion) UV protection is vital. Any unprotected exposure to the sun can erase weeks' worth of consistent efforts.

Another method that may be used in conjunction with a lightening product is microdermabrasion. Microdermabrasion is a process in which a thin layer of skin is removed in a series of sessions. A device sprays a miniature stream of an abrasive material that is immediately suctioned off the skin with a light vacuum. All of this occurs in one sweeping motion of a small wand attachment progressively covering the area to be treated. The procedure removes a very thin layer of the epidermis. When carried out in a series of six to eight treatments (with hyperpigmentation it is not uncommon to go several treatments beyond this initial series), the results are a smoother more even-toned complexion. Darker areas become lighter due to the removal of the layers. Other benefits of microdermabrasion include an increase in cellular renewal, and there is no down time with the treatment. The procedure may take forty-five minutes to an hour depending on the area treated and can cost anywhere from $100–$200 and up. Most salons or dermatologists will give a discounted price for the procedure if purchased as a series. Great strides in improving the complexion can be seen when partnering microdermabrasion and a good botanical treatment. Products can more readily penetrate the epidermis because layers of skin and dead cells have been removed and no longer inhibit or slow absorption. Whatever method is chosen by the client and therapist, UV protection must always be observed on a daily basis, rain or shine. Treating hyperpigmentation is a progressive and cooperative effort. Results will not be realized immediately; again, patience and consistence will bring about the desired results if the condition is treatable. Be sure that the skin care therapist is one that you are comfortable with and is knowledgeable about working with skin of color.

Last, but not least, some discoloration on the skin is not caused by any of these factors, but simply comes from a lack of proper cleansing and skin hygiene. All product lines are not created equal. At the beginning of this book, we discussed a customized skin care routine. Proper removal of dead skin and oils from the skin will result in a more clear, even-toned, and healthy complexion. It is definitely worth seeking professional advice to obtain products suitable to your needs. When proper instruction is given and good cleansing habits are performed, the world will take notice.

BECAUSE I'M WORTH IT!

Do you complain about the way your skin looks but don't do anything about it? *If you've read this far, you'd better be working on doing something about it!* Do you complain about how the products you buy at the drugstore don't work, yet you keep buying those same drugstore products? Do you complain about blemishes, dryness, rough skin, spots, acne, but don't seek any advice on what to do for those conditions? Wake up! Your skin is pleading for help, and you're not listening.

We've covered so much ground. What does it take to show yourself that you appreciate you? You owe it to yourself to stay in good health, to eat right and exercise, to care for your personal well-being. If you don't who will? One body, one you. You may be able to trade in a few pieces for a larger/smaller size, or have something sucked out, cut off, dyed, plucked out, or whatever, but you can't buy another skin. Your best bet is to value who you are, not out of vanity, but out of respect for yourself. You are worth investing in.

Purchasing goods and services for personal wellness is making an investment in you. Seeking out professional expertise increases your knowledge on how to better care for yourself and saves you money in the long run.

Going to the Spa

Let's say you've decided you can't live with the breakout you continue to have from month to month. Your over-the-counter cleanser you've been using for the last three years just doesn't seem to be doing anything or may be contributing to the problem. A visit to the office of a professional skin therapist can save you considerable frustration. How? This is worth repeating—go back to the chapter "Why Customized Skin Care Is Important!" A good therapist will consult with you and examine your skin. Through her observations and questions to you, she'll be able to help you determine the best course of action to combat your skin condition. You can discuss product ingredients to see if what you're using is in fact working contrary to your goals. If need be, she'll refer you to a dermatologist for medical help.

Your initial investment may be between $70–$95 for a consultation and facial lower or higher depending on where you live. If you purchase professional skin care products you may spend another $60–$250. Everyone wants nice, clear skin. Some of us will have to work at it a little harder than others.

One of the most pleasing and usually tremendously enjoyable things in life is to have someone pamper and spoil you. Whether it's going shopping, out to dinner or movie, or getting your nails done, when someone else treats you special, you feel on top of the world. Going to a skin care center or spa is just as wonderful as any of these things. You can receive services ranging from facials to body wraps. You can sip soothing herbal teas and fruit waters while listening to the sound of music played ever so softly. Or perhaps, a facial is in order with an esthetic massage to the rhythmic sounds of crashing waves or gentle rain. Purely pampering? Absolutely not! The best part of all is that you can relax while receiving beneficial treatments that feel good, smell good, and do a world of good for your skin. Menu selections at skin care centers and spas are as varied as the many restaurant menus in any city. Stop by and visit those in your area or nearby. Try to go to more than one. Some have interesting themes associated with their treatments and centers. Gather several menus and peruse for treatments that interest you. This is a good way to make a cost comparison also. Ask friends or coworkers that have visited one or two for recommendations. Wherever you decide to go for your treatment or therapy, you should feel comfortable about the spa itself, and the skin care therapist that will assist you that day. If there is anything you are uncomfortable with, do not hesitate to make it known. Your enjoyment is contingent upon you're being at ease, otherwise, you won't be able to relax during the treatment.

When visiting, check for cleanliness of staff and facility. Most states have a rating system for sanitation; look for this rating and hope it's in the high 90s or 100, or grade A. This way, you'll know the people you are dealing with care about their clientele and health issues. It's not a bad idea either to ask them if they are experienced in and comfortable in working with skin of color. Hey, unfortunately, not all grass is green and even though someone is supposed to be a professional, they may not be as informed or comfortable when addressing this issue. If this is the case, you have the option of walking away. Sometimes, even when the grass is green, you still have to walk away. The more prepared you are, the more you'll know whether they aren't.

Specialized Treatments

Are you throwing your money away? Of course not! Sometimes you just can't skimp when it comes to reaching your personal goals. Does this mean that you spend beyond your means? Certainly not! But it does mean that you should make every effort to do the best that you can for yourself in everything. Don't sell yourself short. High dollar doesn't necessarily equate to high maintenance, but rather to quality in services and efficacy in product.

A company known for its best-selling hair-color product has its spokeswoman asks its consumers "Why?" (does she use the hair coloring?) and then she responds, "Because I'm worth it." When you feel good about yourself, you project a positive image to others.

One of the great things about skin care is that you can choose how far you want to go with it. There are noninvasive procedures that will rejuvenate the skin and accelerate cellular production to produce younger looking, more vibrant skin. Procedures can be customized to help reduce the appearance of hyperpigmentation and even out the complexion and some to combat acne and help reduce blemishes.

A trip to the spa no matter how often you get to go is an experience that can benefit everyone. For instance, young women in their teens would benefit greatly from a basic sort of facial that caters to gentle cleansing of delicate skin to help prevent blemishes. If the teen already is suffering from acne or breakout, a facial customized to deeply but gently cleanse the pores, reduce inflammation, and calm the skin could be the order for the day. At an early age they are taught proper cleansing and hygiene techniques to keep their skin looking good and to continue to take care of it for a lifetime.

As early as the twenties we begin to start experiencing signs of aging even if they are not evident yet. The days spent out of doors without protection, begin their cumulative affect in the sub layers of our skin. Preventative facial therapies are excellent to help keep the skin vibrant and protected.

Specialized serums loaded with antioxidants and vitamins are essential to waylay the effects of environmental stresses.

At our thirties and forties we begin to see definite signs of aging as the skin loses some of its vibrancy and fine lines try to come on the scene. At the spa these traumas can be addressed with rejuvenating facial therapy that focuses on removal of dead skin, nourishing the skin with potent vitamins such as vitamin C, maintaining hydration and protecting the skin from further damage as much as possible.

Toward our fifties and beyond, revitalizing therapies are a wonderful way to battles stress around the eyes where wrinkles tend to gather. Therapies that address attention to maintaining balance of oil and moisture to alleviate dry tight skin are needed due to increased hormonal changes. Vitamin and antioxidant therapy is also a plus and can be combined with other modalities. Microdermabrasion or resurfacing therapies help to kick the skin into gear to produce new healthy cells, maintain a more even complexion and to smooth the skin, resulting in a more youthful appearance. (*And who doesn't want to look more youthful?*)

Whether skin care, hair coloring, nail services, or a professional trainer for fitness, every dollar invested in you is money well spent. It is within your power to control the gains and losses of your personal wellness investment. You have to calculate the risks (if any) and analyze the potential for growth (in self-esteem, personal wellness, self-worth, etc.). If you don't think enough of yourself to invest in you, why should others? Know that you are valuable and worthy to do and receive things that make you feel good about who you are! Phenomenal skin begins with phenomenal care!

I LEAVE YOU WITH THESE THOUGHTS

My mom, many years ago, asked me a profound question that I continue to dwell on from time to time. I was going through a particularly *ugly* period in my life. I felt that I would never look as good as many of my classmates. I was too short, not very well endowed, sort of blending in with the woodwork. I was not popular. The guys I liked only liked the beautiful people. Unfortunately, that followed me into my adult life, and I always seemed to feel inferior to other women, especially those I considered beautiful. She said to me, "Terry, if you never believe you look good, then why should anyone else?" Was she giving me a license to be vain and conceited? Certainly not, but in her characteristically direct manner was only trying to help me understand that I must believe that I am of great value and never allow anyone to diminish that; to not let my happiness, my self-esteem, or my dreams be contingent upon what others believe or say about me. Most importantly, I am never to compare myself to anyone else. I am responsible for defining who I am. She led me to always rely on Christ because only he could bring out the true beauty within me. My mom is the most beautiful woman in the world. Thanks, Mom!

Society dictates that real beauty looks a certain way, has a certain body shape, skin/hair color, hair texture, graces the cover of only the most prestigious publications, etc. We spend so much time and money getting things altered, enhanced, reshaped, and removed to live up to those standards that sometimes we lose sight of who we really are. There is nothing at all wrong with pursuing these things, but just remember that you are already marvelously made. Yes, we should definitely take care of what God has given us, whether taking care of our skin or keeping our bodies fit. We should invest in ourselves; it is neither selfish nor vain because we never forget that we are truly fearfully and wonderfully made and as such always beautiful and precious in our Lord's sight.

PERSONAL SKIN JOURNAL

Personal promise to myself:

I will do what is necessary to change my current skin condition. It is up to me to take action to reach my desired goal. I realize that consistency and patience will be key factors to my achieving my goal. I endeavor to invest the time, money and effort in myself to accomplish my goal because I am worth it.

Name ———————————————— Date ————————

The purpose of this journal is to keep track of my personal skin care journey. In it, I record my purchases, thoughts on my therapies received, and any questions I may have about my skin that I want to share with my therapist. I can also record any breakout occurrences, stressful situations and periods in my life, and all progress toward the finish line of clear skin, an even complexion, high self-esteem, and faith in myself as a lovely, beautiful, godly, and intelligent individual.

I believe my skin condition to be ————————————
(refer to the chapter "What about Me?").

Confirmed by therapist/esthetician? Yes/No

Budget for skin care (includes therapy and products)
$ ————— /month

Top three products I've researched (try to study at least four or five and pick the three best ones you are impressed with. If that's too confusing, stick with three.)

Brand Name	Active Ingredients	Possible Allergens?	Price Points $ $	In budget?	Samples available?	Professional or over the ctn.

Final Product Selection:
Brand Name: _____

Therapies: _____

Cleanser	Toner	Masque	Exfoliant
Hydrator/Moisturizer	Sun/Solar Care		
Specialty:	Serums	Eye Treatment	Blemish Control

DAILY WORK SHEET

Date _____

This is my daily log to record my progress in reaching my skin care goals, my everyday successes, my temporary setbacks, my venue for venting, and moving on!

This is the day that the Lord has made, I will rejoice and be glad in it!

Skin Log (Record any changes in your skin or the addition of a new therapy, etc.):

_____

_____

_____

_____

_____

_____

_____

_____

My Daily Post

_____

_____

_____

_____

_____

_____

_____

_____

_____

_____

_____

_____

_____

_____

_____

_____

_____

_____

_____

_____

_____

_____

_____

What can I do to change my reactive responses to a more positive response to circumstances?

_____

_____

_____